A PRACTICAL HANDBOOK

Third Edition 2012

GW00702432

MANAGEMENT OF SEVERE MALARIA

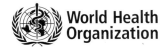
World Health Organization

WHO Library Cataloguing-in-Publication Data

Management of severe malaria: a practical handbook – 3rd ed.

　　1.Malaria – complications. 2.Malaria – drug therapy.
　　3.Handbooks. I.World Health Organization.

　　ISBN 978 92 4 154852 6　　　　　　　　NLM classification: WC 39)

Please consult the WHO Global Malaria Programme web site for the
most up-to-date version of all documents (www.who.int/malaria).

Printed in Italy
Design by Paprika-annecy.com

TABLE OF CONTENTS

PREFACE 3

INTRODUCTION 5

SEVERE FALCIPARUM MALARIA 7

SEVERE VIVAX MALARIA 9

SEVERE KNOWLESI MALARIA 10

DIAGNOSIS OF MALARIA 11

GENERAL MANAGEMENT 15

NURSING CARE 19

● CLINICAL FEATURES OF SEVERE MALARIA AND
  MANAGEMENT OF COMMON COMPLICATIONS IN
  CHILDREN 23

  Severe malaria 23
  Cerebral malaria 28
  Anaemia 33
  Respiratory distress (acidosis) 36
  Hypoglycaemia 37
  Shock 38
  Dehydration and electrolyte disturbance 39
  Children unable to retain oral medication 41
  Post discharge follow-up of children with severe malaria 41
  Antimalarial drugs 41

● CLINICAL FEATURES OF SEVERE MALARIA AND
  MANAGEMENT OF COMPLICATIONS IN ADULTS 43

  Cerebral malaria 43
  Anaemia 46
  Acute kidney injury 46
  Hypoglycaemia 48
  Metabolic acidosis 49
  Pulmonary oedema 50
  Shock 52

Abnormal bleeding and disseminated intravascular coagulation 53
Haemoglobinuria 54
Antimalarial drugs 54

⬤ SPECIAL CLINICAL FEATURES AND MANAGEMENT
OF SEVERE MALARIA IN PREGNANCY 55
   Severe malaria 55
   Hypoglycaemia 56
   Pulmonary oedema 57
   Anaemia 58
   Antimalarial drugs 58

⬤ PROGNOSTIC INDICATORS IN SEVERE
FALCIPARUM MALARIA 59

⬤ COMMON ERRORS IN DIAGNOSIS AND MANAGEMENT 61
   Errors in diagnosis 61
   Errors in management 62

ANNEX 1. SELECTED FURTHER READING 65
ANNEX 2. MEMBERS OF THE REVIEW COMMITTEE 66
ANNEX 3. PERFORMING AND INTERPRETING RAPID
          DIAGNOSTIC TESTS 69
ANNEX 4. NOTES ON ANTIMALARIAL DRUGS 72
ANNEX 5. COMA SCALES 74
          5a. Blantyre coma scale for children 74
          5b. The Glasgow coma scale (for adults and children >5 years) 75
ANNEX 6. SETTING UP AN INTRA-OSSEOUS INFUSION
          FOR CHILDREN 76
ANNEX 7. MEASURING JUGULAR VENOUS PRESSURE 79
ANNEX 8. PERITONEAL DIALYSIS 81
ANNEX 9. CALCULATING VOLUMES OF MAINTENANCE
          FLUIDS AND BLOOD TRANSFUSIONS 83

PREFACE

Malaria continues to be a major global health problem, with over 40% of the world's population—more than 3.3 billion people—at risk for malaria to varying degrees in countries with on-going transmission. In addition, with modern, rapid means of travel, large numbers of people from non-malarious areas are being infected, which may seriously affect them after they have returned home. During the past decade, investments in malaria prevention and control have created unparalleled momentum and saved more than 1 million lives. The rates of death from malaria have been cut by over one fourth worldwide and by one third in the World Health Organization (WHO) African Region. Malaria transmission still occurs, however, in 99 countries, and the disease caused an estimated 655 000 deaths in 2010 (with an uncertainty range of 537 000–907 000 deaths), mainly among children under 5 years of age in sub-Saharan Africa.[1]

Plasmodium falciparum is common in the tropics and causes the most serious form of the disease. Infections with this parasite can be fatal in the absence of prompt recognition of the disease and its complications and urgent, appropriate patient management. *P. vivax* and *P. knowlesi* (a species that primarily infects monkeys and may be transmitted to humans in certain forested areas of South-East Asia) may also cause severe infections. Resistance of parasites to antimalaria agents continues to be a threat to malaria control and elimination efforts globally. The emergence of resistance to artemisinins in the Mekong sub-Region is of particular concern. Prompt diagnosis and treatment

---

1 *World malaria report 2011*. Geneva, World Health Organization, 2011. http://www. who.int/malaria/world_malaria_report_2011/9789241564403_eng.pdf.

are crucial to prevent mortality, especially in high-risk groups such as young children and pregnant women.

This practical handbook on the management of severe and complicated malaria has been revised and updated for the third time, with some key changes, notably, replacement of quinine with artesunate as first-line treatment for severe malaria caused by all *Plasmodium* species. Like previous editions, this handbook is intended primarily for health professionals working in hospitals or health centres with inpatient facilities, who are responsible for the management of patients with severe malaria. As this manual focuses on the practical management of severe malaria, it is based on guidelines and recommendations adopted as standard WHO guidance for the management of severe malaria or severely ill patients, which are listed in Annex 1. When new information or a new recommendation that has not previously been endorsed in a WHO guideline is given, the source of the information or the basis of the recommendation is referenced. The review of the handbook was organised through a consultation of the GMP Technical Expert Group (TEG) on Malaria Chemotherapy co-chaired by Professors Fred Binka and Nick White (Annex 2).

The WHO Global Malaria Programme would like to thank Medicines for Malaria Venture (MMV), Roll Back Malaria (Case Management Working Group), and the UK Department for International Development (DFID), for providing financial support to the development and production of this manual.

INTRODUCTION

Severe malaria is most commonly caused by infection with *Plasmodium falciparum*, although *P. vivax* and *P. knowlesi*[2,3] can also cause severe disease. The risk is increased if treatment of an uncomplicated attack of malaria caused by these parasites is delayed. Recognizing and promptly treating uncomplicated malaria is therefore of vital importance. Sometimes, however, especially in children, severe *P. falciparum* malaria may develop so rapidly that early treatment of uncomplicated malaria is not feasible.

The presentation of uncomplicated *P. falciparum* malaria is highly variable and mimics that of many other diseases. Although fever is common, it is often intermittent and may even be absent in some cases. The fever is typically irregular initially and commonly associated with chills. True rigors are unusual in acute falciparum malaria. The patient commonly complains of fever, headache, aches and pains elsewhere in the body and occasionally abdominal pain and diarrhoea. In a young child, there may be irritability, refusal to eat and vomiting. On physical examination, fever may be the only sign. In some patients, the liver and spleen are palpable. This clinical presentation is usually indistinguishable clinically from those of influenza and a variety of other common causes of fever. Unless the condition is diagnosed and treated promptly, a patient with falciparum malaria may deteriorate rapidly.

2   Cox-Singh J et al. (2008). *Plasmodium knowlesi* malaria in humans is widely distributed and potentially life threatening. *Clinical Infectious Diseases*, 46:165–171.
3   Kantele A, Jokiranta S (2011) Review of cases with the emerging fifth human malaria parasite, *Plasmodium knowlesi. Clinical Infectious Diseases*, 52:1356–1362.

SEVERE FALCIPARUM MALARIA

Malaria infections may cause vital organ dysfunction and death. Severe malaria is defined by clinical or laboratory evidence of vital organ dysfunction. Nearly all deaths from severe malaria result from infections with *P. falciparum*. Strict definitions of severe malaria have been published for epidemiological and research purposes, but, in practice, there should be a low threshold for starting parenteral treatment in any patient about whom a health care worker is concerned. Even if some of the laboratory measures are not available immediately, this should not delay the start of intensive treatment.

A general overview of the features of severe malaria is shown in the box below. Note that these manifestations can occur singly or, more commonly, in combination in the same patient.

Clinical features of severe malaria

- impaired consciousness (including unrousable coma);
- prostration, i.e. generalized weakness so that the patient is unable to sit, stand or walk without assistance;
- multiple convulsions: more than two episodes within 24h;
- deep breathing and respiratory distress (acidotic breathing);
- acute pulmonary oedema and acute respiratory distress syndrome;
- circulatory collapse or shock, systolic blood pressure < 80mm Hg in adults and < 50mm Hg in children;
- acute kidney injury;
- clinical jaundice plus evidence of other vital organ dysfunction; and
- abnormal bleeding.

High parasitaemia is undoubtedly a risk factor for death from falciparum malaria, but the relation between parasitaemia and prognosis varies according to the level of malaria transmission. In low-transmission areas, mortality from acute falciparum malaria begins to increase with parasite densities over 100 000/µl (~2.5% parasitaemia), whereas in areas of higher transmission much higher parasite densities may be well tolerated. Parasitaemia > 20% is associated with a high risk in any epidemiological context.

Laboratory and other findings

- hypoglycaemia (< 2.2mmol/l or < 40mg/dl);
- metabolic acidosis (plasma bicarbonate < 15mmol/l);
- severe normocytic anaemia (haemoglobin < 5g/dl, packed cell volume < 15% in children; <7g/dl, packed cell volume < 20% in adults);
- haemoglobinuria;
- hyperlactataemia (lactate > 5mmol/l);
- renal impairment (serum creatinine > 265µmol/l); and
- pulmonary oedema (radiological).

Who is at risk?

In high-transmission areas, the risk for severe falciparum malaria is greatest among young children and visitors (of any age) from nonendemic areas. In other areas, severe malaria is more evenly distributed across all age groups. Risk is increased in the second and third trimesters of pregnancy, in patients with HIV/AIDS and in people who have undergone splenectomy.

- High transmission area: hyperendemic or holoendemic area in which the prevalence rate of *P. falciparum* parasitaemia is over 50% most of the year among children aged 2–9 years. In these areas, virtually all exposed individuals have been infected by late infancy or early childhood.
- Moderate transmission area: mesoendemic area in which the prevalence rate of *P. falciparum* parasitaemia is 11–50% during most of the year among children aged 2–9 years. The maximum prevalence of malaria occurs in childhood and adolescence, although it is not unusual for adulthood to be attained before an infection is acquired.
- Low transmission area: hypoendemic area in which the prevalence rate of *P. falciparum* parasitaemia is 10% or less during most of the year among children aged 2–9 years. Malaria infection and disease may occur at a similarly low frequency at any age, as little immunity develops and people may go through life without being infected.

SEVERE VIVAX MALARIA

P. vivax infection is much less likely to progress to severe malaria than *P. falciparum* infection. Severe vivax malaria may present with some symptoms similar to those of severe *P. falciparum* malaria and can be fatal. Severe anaemia and respiratory distress occur at all ages, although severe anaemia is particularly common in young children.

Who is at risk?

The risk for severe vivax malaria is greatest among young children and people with comorbid conditions. Severe disease is rare in temperate areas and in returned travellers. It occurs in relatively high-transmission areas with chloroquine resistance, such as Indonesia and Papua New Guinea, as well as in low-transmission areas, including India and South America.

SEVERE KNOWLESI MALARIA

The monkey parasite *P. knowlesi* can cause malaria in humans living in close proximity to macaque monkeys (particularly on the island of Borneo). Under the microscope, mature parasites are indistinguishable from those of *P. malariae* and are commonly diagnosed as such. Ring stages resemble those of *P. falciparum*. *P. knowlesi* replicates every 24h, which can result in rapidly increasing parasite densities, severe disease and death in some individuals. The severe manifestations are similar to those of severe falciparum malaria, with the exception of coma. Early diagnosis and treatment are therefore essential. In Asia, patients with *P. malariae* like infections and unusually high parasite densities (parasitaemia > 0.5% by microscopy) should be managed in the same way as for *P. knowlesi* infection. A definitive diagnosis is made by polymerase chain reaction.

Who is at risk?

P. knowlesi malaria occurs mainly on the island of Borneo but has been reported in other South-East Asian countries. Local residents and travellers to or from this region are at risk for infection. It is transmitted mainly in forests and along forest fringes.

Clinical diagnosis

The most important element in the clinical diagnosis of malaria, in both endemic and non-endemic areas, is a high index of suspicion. Because the distribution of malaria is patchy, even in countries where it is prevalent, information on residence and travel history indicative of exposure is important. In addition, the possibility of induced malaria (through transfusion or use of contaminated needles) must not be overlooked.

Severe malaria can mimic many other diseases that are also common in malaria-endemic countries. The most important of these are central nervous system infections, septicaemia, severe pneumonia and typhoid fever. Other differential diagnoses include influenza, dengue and other arbovirus infections, hepatitis, leptospirosis, the relapsing fevers, haemorrhagic fevers, rickettsial infections, gastroenteritis and, in Africa, trypanosomiasis.

In children, convulsions due to malaria must be differentiated from febrile convulsions. In the latter, post-ictal coma usually lasts no longer than half an hour, although some children do not regain full consciousness until 60min after a seizure.

Parasitological diagnosis of severe falciparum malaria

Microscopy is the gold standard and preferred option for diagnosing malaria. In nearly all cases, examination of thick and thin blood films will reveal malaria parasites. Thick films are more sensitive than thin films for detecting low-density malaria parasitaemia (Figures 1 and 2). Facilities and equipment for microscopic examination of blood films can be set up easily in a side-room of a clinic or ward, and films can be read by trained personnel on site. This reduces the delay that commonly occurs when samples must be sent to a distant laboratory. In general, the greater the parasite density in the peripheral blood, the higher the likelihood that severe disease is present or will develop, especially among 'non-immune' patients. Nevertheless, as the parasites in severe falciparum malaria are usually sequestered in capillaries and venules (and therefore not seen on a peripheral blood slide), patients may present with severe malaria with very low peripheral parasitaemia. Where microscopy is unavailable or unfeasible, a rapid diagnostic test (RDT) should be used. RDTs for detecting *HRP2* antigen can be useful for diagnosing malaria in patients who have recently received antimalarial treatment and in whom blood films are transiently negative for malaria parasites. Rarely, the blood film is negative in a patient who dies and is found at autopsy to have intense tissue sequestration of *P. falciparum*. If both the slide and the RDT are negative, the patient is extremely unlikely to have malaria, and other causes of illness should be sought and treated. Frequent monitoring of parasitaemia (e.g. every 12h) is important during the first 2–3 days of treatment in order to monitor the parasite response to the antimalarial medicine. This is particularly important in South-East Asia where artemisinin resistance is emerging.

RDTs for detecting *PfHRP2* antigen cannot be used to monitor the response to treatment, as they can remain positive for up to 4 weeks after clearance of parasitaemia. None of the RDTs currently on the market provides information on parasite density or the stage of malaria parasites, which are important parameters in monitoring a patient being treated for severe malaria (see Annex 3).

Figure 1: Species identification of malaria parasites in Giemsa- stained thick blood film

Species		Trophozoite	Schizont	Gametocyte
Plasmodium falciparum	Young, growing trophozoites and/or mature gametocytes usually seen	**Size**: small to medium; **number**: often numerous; **shape**: ring and comma forms common; **chromatin**: often two dots; cytoplasm: regular, fine to fleshy; **mature forms**: sometimes present in severe malaria, compact with **pigment** as few coarse grains or a mass	Usually associated with many young ring forms. **Size**: small, compact,; **number**: few, uncommon, usually in severe malaria; **mature forms**: 12-30 or more merozoites in compact cluster; **pigment**: single dark mass	Immature pointed-end forms uncommon. **mature forms**: banana-shaped or rounded: **chromatin**: single, well defined; **pigment**: scattered, coarse, rice-grain-like; pink extrusion body sometimes present. Eroded forms with only chromatin and pigment often seen.
Plasmodium vivax	All stages seen; Schüffner stippling in 'ghost' of host red cells, especially at film edge	**Size**: small to large; **number**: few to moderate; **shape**: broken ring to irregular forms common; **chromatin**: single, occasionally two; cytoplasm: irregular or fragmented; **mature forms**: compact, dense; **pigment**: scattered, fine	**Size**: large; **number**: few to moderate, **mature forms**: 12-24 merozoites, usually 16, in irregular cluster; **pigment**: loose mass	Immature forms difficult to distinguish from mature trophozoites. **mature forms**: round, large; **chromatin**: single, well defined; **pigment**: scattered, fine. Eroded forms with scanty or no cytoplasm and only chromatin and pigment present.
Plasmodium ovale	All stages seen; prominent Schüffner stippling in 'ghost' of host red cells, especially at film edge	**Size**: may be smaller than *P. vivax*; **number**: usually few; **shape**: ring to rounded, compact forms; **chromatin**: single, prominent; cytoplasm: fairly regular, fleshy; **pigment**: scattered, coarse.	Immature forms difficult to distinguish from mature trophozoites. **mature forms**: round, may be smaller than *P. vivax*; **chromatin**: single, well defined; **pigment**: scattered, coarse. Eroded forms with only chromatin and pigment present.	**Size**: rather like *P. malariae*; **number**: few; **mature forms**: 4-12 merozoites, usually 8, in loose cluster; **pigment**: concentrated mass.
Plasmodium malariae	All stages seen	**Size**: small: usually few; **shape**: ring to rounded, compact forms; **chromatin**: single, large; cytoplasm: regular, dense; **pigment**: scattered, abundant, with yellow tinge in older forms.	**Size**: small, compact; **number**: usually few; **mature forms**: 6-12 merozoites, usually 8, in loose cluster, some apparently without cytoplasm; **pigment**: concentrated.	Immature and certain **mature forms** difficult to distinguish from mature trophozoites. **mature forms**: round, compact; **chromatin**: single, well defined; **pigment**: scattered, coarse, may be peripherally distributed. Eroded forms with only chromatin and pigment present.

Parasitological diagnosis of severe vivax and knowlesi malaria

In the clinical setting, microscopy is the gold standard for detecting malaria and identifying the species of plasmodium involved. The currently available RDTs are slightly less sensitive for detecting *P. vivax* than for *P. falciparum*. As *P. knowlesi* and *P. malariae* are similar, microscopy alone is insufficient to diagnose *P. knowlesi*. A high parasite density (> 0.5% parasitaemia) with *P. malariae*-like parasites should be treated for *P. knowlesi* infection. Polymerase chain reaction is required to confirm *P. knowlesi* infection, but should not delay treatment.

Haematological and biochemical findings in severe malaria

Anaemia is normocytic and may be 'severe' (haemoglobin < 5g/dl or erythrocyte volume fraction (haematocrit) < 15%. Thrombocytopenia (< 100 000 platelets/µl) is usual in malaria, and in some cases the platelet count may be extremely low (< 20 000/µl). Polymorphonuclear leukocytosis is found in some patients with the most severe disease. Serum or plasma concentrations of urea, creatinine, bilirubin and liver and muscle enzymes (e.g. aminotransferases and 5'-nucleotidase, creatine phosphokinase) may be elevated, although the levels of liver enzymes are much lower than in acute viral hepatitis. Severely ill patients are commonly acidotic, with low plasma pH and bicarbonate concentrations. Electrolyte disturbances (sodium, potassium, chloride, calcium and phosphate) may occur.

Figure 2: **Appearance of *P. falciparum* parasite stages in Giemsa-stained thin and thick blood films**

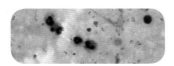 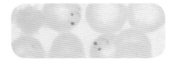

GENERAL MANAGEMENT

The following measures should be taken for all patients with clinically diagnosed or suspected severe malaria:

- Make a rapid clinical assessment, with special attention to the general condition and level of consciousness, blood pressure, rate and depth of respiration and pallor. Assess neck stiffness and examine for rash to exclude alternative diagnoses.

- Admit the patient to an acute illness ward or room; or next to the nurses' station in a general ward for close monitoring. However if indicated and available, admit the patient to an intensive care unit.

- Make a rapid initial check of the blood glucose level, correct hypoglycaemia if present, and then monitor frequently for hypoglycaemia.

- If possible, examine the optic fundi. Retinal whitening, vascular changes or haemorrhages, if present, will help diagnosis. The examination will rarely reveal papilloedema, which is a contraindication to a lumbar puncture (Figure 3).

- Treat seizures with a benzodiazepine (intravenous diazepam, midazolam or lorazepam). If a seizure episode persists longer than 10min after the first dose, give a second dose of a benzodiazepine (diazepam, midazolam or lorazepam).[4] Seizures that persist (status epilepticus) despite the use of two doses of these drugs present a difficult problem. For such cases, give phenytoin

---

4   The total dose of benzodiazepine should not exceed 1mg/kg within a 24-h period.

18mg/kg body weight intravenously, or phenobarbitone 15mg/kg body weight intramuscularly or intravenously if it is the only available option. Monitor breathing repeatedly, as a high dose of phenobarbitone (20mg/kg body weight) has been linked to an increased risk for death[5] and the patient may need assisted ventilation.

- If parasitological confirmation of malaria is not readily feasible, make a blood film and start treatment for severe malaria on the basis of the clinical presentation.

- Give artesunate intravenously. If artesunate is not available give intramuscular artemether or intravenous quinine. If intravenous administration is not possible, artesunate or quinine may be given intramuscularly into the anterior thigh. Suppository formulations of artemisinin and its derivatives should be given as pre-referral treatment where parenteral therapy with artesunate or quinine is not possible or feasible.

- Give parenteral antimalarial agents in the treatment of severe malaria for a minimum of 24h, even if the patient is able to tolerate oral medication earlier. Thereafter, give a full course of the oral artemisinin-based combination therapy that is effective in the area where the infection was acquired.

5   Crawley J et al. (2000). Effect of phenobarbital on seizure frequency and mortality in childhood cerebral malaria: a randomized controlled intervention study. Lancet, 355:701–706.

- Calculate the dose of artesunate, artemether or quinine as mg/kg of body weight. All patients should be weighed; if this is not possible, the patient's weight should be estimated.

- Provide good nursing care. This is vital, especially if the patient is unconscious (see page 19).

- Pay careful attention to the patient's fluid balance in severe malaria in order to avoid over- or underhydration. Individual requirements vary widely, depending on fluid losses before admission. Children with severe malaria who are unable to retain oral fluids should be managed with 5% dextrose and / isotonic saline (0.9%) maintenance fluids (3-4ml/kg/hour), and adults at 1-2ml/kg body weight per hour, until the patient is able to take and retain oral fluids. Rapid fluid boluses are contraindicated in severe malaria resuscitation. Dehydration should be managed cautiously and ideally guided by urine output (with a urine output goal of > 1ml/kg body weight per hour), unless the patient has anuric renal failure or pulmonary oedema, for which fluid management should be tailored to the needs of the patient and reassessed frequently.

- Make sure to look for other treatable causes of coma. Meningitis should be excluded by lumbar puncture. If lumbar puncture is contraindicated or not feasible, the patient should receive presumptive antibiotic treatment (see page 21).

- Look for and manage any other complicating or associated infections.

- Record urine output, and look for the appearance of brown or black urine (haemoglobinuria) or oliguria, which may indicate acute kidney injury.

- Monitor the therapeutic response, both clinical and parasitological, by regular observation and blood films.

- Monitor the core temperature (preferably rectal), respiratory rate and depth, pulse, blood pressure and level of consciousness regularly. These observations will allow identification of complications such as hypoglycaemia, metabolic acidosis (indicated by the presence or development of deep breathing), pulmonary oedema and hypotensive shock. In children, a capillary refill time of > 2s, often associated with other signs of impaired perfusion, defines a high-risk group that should be monitored closely.

- Reduce high body temperatures (> 39°C) by administering paracetamol as an antipyretic. Tepid sponging and fanning may make the patient comfortable.

- Carry out regular laboratory evaluation of erythrocyte volume fraction (haematocrit) or haemoglobin concentration, glucose, urea or creatinine and electrolytes.

- Avoid drugs that increase the risk for gastrointestinal bleeding (aspirin, corticosteroids).

- More sophisticated monitoring (e.g. measurement of arterial pH, blood gases) may be useful if complications develop; this will depend on the local availability of equipment, experience and skills.

Figure 3: **Retinopathy in a child with cerebral malaria.**

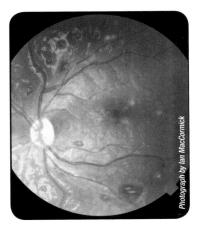

Photograph by Ian MacCormick

Note the characteristic patchy retinal whitening around the fovea (~3 disc-diameters to the right of the optic disc). Note also some white-centred haemorrhages.

NURSING CARE

Good nursing care of patients with severe malaria is of vital importance.

- Ensure meticulous nursing care. This can be life-saving, especially for unconscious patients. Maintain a clear airway. Nurse the patient in the lateral or semi-prone position to avoid aspiration of fluid. If the patient is unconscious, insert a nasogastric tube and aspirate the stomach contents to minimize the risk for aspiration pneumonia, which is a potentially fatal complication that must be dealt with immediately.

- Turn the patient every 2h. Do not allow the patient to lie in a wet bed. Pay particular attention to pressure points.

- Suspect raised intracranial pressure in patients with irregular respiration, abnormal posturing, worsening coma, unequal or dilated pupils, elevated blood pressure and falling heart rate, or papilloedema. In all such cases, nurse the patient in a supine posture with the head of the bed raised.

- Keep a careful record of fluid intake and output. If this is not possible, weigh the patient daily to calculate the approximate fluid balance. All patients who are unable to take oral fluids should receive dextrose-containing maintenance fluids, unless contraindicated (fluid overload), until they are able to drink and retain fluids. Check the speed of infusion of fluids frequently: too fast or too slow an infusion can be dangerous.

- Monitor the temperature, pulse, respiration, blood pressure and level of consciousness (use a paediatric scale for children and the Glasgow coma scale for adults; see Annex 5). These observations should be made at least every 4h until the patient is out of danger.

- Report deterioration of the level of consciousness, occurrence of convulsions or changes in behaviour of the patient immediately. All such changes suggest developments that require additional treatment.

- If the rectal temperature rises above 39°C, remove the patient's clothes, give oral or rectal paracetamol and make the child comfortable with tepid sponging and fanning.

- Note any appearance of red or black urine (haemoglobinuria). For all such patients, determine the blood group, cross-match blood ready for transfusion if necessary and increase the frequency of haematocrit assessment, as severe anaemia may develop rapidly. In this situation, the haematocrit is a better measure than the haemoglobin concentration, because the latter quantifies not only haemoglobin in red cells but also free plasma haemoglobin.

Specific antimalarial chemotherapy

The recommended treatment for severe malaria is intravenous artesunate (see inside front cover flap). Information on the most commonly used medicines is given in Annex 4.

Antibiotics

There is considerable clinical overlap between septicaemia, pneumonia and severe malaria, and these conditions may coexist. In malaria-endemic areas, particularly where parasitaemia is common in young people, it is often impossible to rule out septicaemia in a severely ill child who is in shock or obtunded. When possible, blood should always be taken on admission for bacterial culture.

Children with suspected severe malaria with associated alterations in the level of consciousness should be started on broad-spectrum antibiotic treatment immediately, at the same time as antimalarial treatment, and treatment should be completed unless a bacterial infection is excluded. In adults with severe malaria, antibiotics are recommended if there is evidence of bacterial co-infection (e.g. hypotension or pneumonia).

CLINICAL FEATURES OF SEVERE MALARIA AND MANAGEMENT OF COMMON COMPLICATIONS IN CHILDREN

SEVERE MALARIA

Clinical features

The commonest, most important complications of *P. falciparum* infection in children are cerebral malaria, severe anaemia, respiratory distress (acidosis) and hypoglycaemia. The differences between severe malaria in adults and in children are shown in Table 1. In all cases of severe malaria, parenteral antimalarial chemotherapy should be started immediately.

History

The parents or other relatives should be questioned about:

- residence and history of travel;
- previous treatment with antimalarial or other drugs;
- recent fluid intake and urine output; and
- recent or history of convulsions.

Initial assessment

The initial assessment of children with severe malaria should include:

- level of consciousness (coma scale for children, Annex 5a);
- evidence of seizures or subtle seizure;
- posturing (decorticate, decerebrate or opisthotonic), which is distinct from seizures;
- rate and depth of respiration;

Table 1: **Signs and symptoms of severe malaria in adults and in children[a]**

Sign or symptom	Adults	Children
Duration of illness	5–7 days	Shorter (1–2 days)
Respiratory distress/ deep breathing (acidosis)	Common	Common
Convulsions	Common (12%)	Very common (30%)
Posturing (decorticate/decerebrate and opisthotonic rigidity)	Uncommon	Common
Prostration/obtundation	Common	Common
Resolution of coma	2–4 days	Faster (1–2 days)
Neurological sequelae after cerebral malaria	Uncommon (1%)	Common (5-30%)
Jaundice	Common	Uncommon
Hypoglycaemia	Less common	Common
Metabolic acidosis	Common	Common
Pulmonary oedema	Uncommon	Rare
Renal failure	Common	Rare
CSF opening pressure	Usually normal	Usually raised
Bleeding/clotting disturbances	Up to 10%	Rare
Invasive bacterial infection (co-infection)	Uncommon (<5%)	Common (10%)

[a] Derived from studies in south-east Asian adults and children, and African children.[6,7]

6   Artesunate vs. quinine in the treatment of severe falciparum malaria in African children (AQUAMAT): an open-label randomized trial. Lancet 2010; 376: 1647–57
7   South-East Asian Quinine Artesunate Malaria Trial (SEAQUAMAT) group. Artesunate versus quinine for treatment of severe falciparum malaria: a randomized Trial. Lancet, 2005, 366:717-725.

- presence of anaemia;
- pulse rate and blood pressure;
- state of hydration;
- capillary refill time; and
- temperature.

Immediate laboratory tests
- thick and thin blood films or RDT if microscopy is not immediately possible or feasible;
- erythrocyte volume fraction (haematocrit);
- blood glucose level; and
- analysis of cerebrospinal fluid (CSF; lumbar puncture).
- blood culture where feasible

Only the results of a lumbar puncture can rule out bacterial meningitis in a child with suspected cerebral malaria. If lumbar puncture is delayed, antibiotics must be given to cover the possibility of bacterial meningitis.

Emergency measures
- Check that the airway is patent; if necessary, provide a Guedel airway for children with seizures.

- Provide oxygen for children with proven or suspected hypoxia (oxygen saturations < 90%). Children at high risk for hypoxia include those with intercurrent seizures (generalized, partial or subtle seizures), children with severe anaemia and those with impaired perfusion (delayed capillary refilling time, weak pulse or cool extremities).

- Provide manual or assisted ventilation with oxygen in case of inadequate breathing.

- Nursing must include all the well-established principles of the care of unconscious children: lay the child in the lateral or semi-prone position, turn them frequently (every 2h) to prevent pressure sores, and provide prospective catheterization to avoid urinary retention and wet bedding. An unconscious child with possible raised intracranial pressure should be nursed in a supine position with the head raised ~30°.

- Correct hypoglycaemia (threshold for intervention: blood glucose < 3mmol/l) with 200 - 500mg/kg of glucose. Immediately give 5ml/kg of 10% dextrose through a peripheral line, and ensure enteral feeding or if not possible maintain with up to 5ml/kg per hour of 10% dextrose. If only 50% dextrose is available, dilute 1 volume of 50% dextrose with 4 volumes sterile water to get 10% dextrose solution (e.g. 0.4ml/kg of 50% dextrose with 1.6ml/kg of water for injection or 4ml of 50% with 16ml of water for injection). Administration of hypertonic glucose (> 20%) is not recommended, as it is an irritant to peripheral veins.

- In any child with convulsions, hyperpyrexia and hypoglycaemia should be excluded.

- Treat convulsions with intravenous diazepam, 0.3mg/kg as a slow bolus ('push') over 2min or 0.5mg/kg of body weight intrarectally. Diazepam may be repeated if seizure activity does not stop after 10min. Midazolam may be used (same dose) instead of diazepam by either the intravenous or buccal route.

- Patients with seizures not terminated by two doses of diazepam should be considered to have status epilepticus and given phenytoin (18mg/kg loading dose, then a maintenance dose of 5mg/kg per day for 48h). If this is not available or fail to control seizures, give phenobarbitone (15mg/kg intramuscularly or slow intravenous loading dose, then a maintenance dose of 5mg/kg per day for 48h). When phenobarbitone is used, monitor the patient's breathing carefully, as it may cause respiratory depression requiring ventilatory support. High-dose (20mg/kg) phenobarbitone may lead to respiratory depression and increased the risk for death. Be prepared to use 'bag-and-mask' manual ventilation if the patient breathes inadequately or to use mechanical ventilation if available.

- Fluid balance maintenance in children who are unable to tolerate or take oral fluids should be by intravenous infusion of fluids at 3–4ml/kg per hour.

- Give a blood transfusion to correct severe anaemia (see page 34).

- Paracetamol at 15mg/kg of body weight every 4h may be given orally or rectally as an antipyretic to keep the rectal temperature below 39°C. Tepid sponging and fanning will make the patient more comfortable.

- Avoid harmful ancillary drugs (see page 45).

Management of the unconscious child

- Clear the airway, check breathing, and provide oxygen. Provide manual or assisted ventilation with oxygen for inadequate breathing.

- Insert a nasogastric tube and, after aspiration, allow free drainage to minimize the risk of aspiration pneumonia.

- Immediate treatment of seizures is important, as prolonged seizures lead to hypoxia and hypercarbia (high pCO_2), which can contribute to or worsen increased intracranial pressure.

- If the child is shown or thought to have raised intracranial pressure, nurse in a supine posture with the head in the midline and with the head of the bed raised 30°.

- Exclude hypoglycaemia and electrolyte imbalance, maintain adequate hydration, and provide dextrose containing maintenance fluids.

- Institute regular observation of vital and neurological signs.

CEREBRAL MALARIA

Clinical features

- The earliest symptom of cerebral malaria in children is usually fever (37.5–41°C), followed by failure to eat or drink. Vomiting and cough are common; diarrhoea is unusual.

- The history of symptoms preceding coma may be brief: commonly 1 or 2 days.

- A child who loses consciousness after a febrile convulsion should not be classified as having cerebral malaria unless the coma persists for more than 30min after the convulsion.

- The depth of coma can be assessed according to the coma scale for children (Annex 5a) by observing the response to standard vocal or painful stimuli (rub knuckles on child's sternum; if there is no response, apply firm horizontal pressure on the thumbnail bed with a pencil). Prostration (inability to sit unsupported in children ≥ 8 months or inability to breastfeed if younger) is a common sign of severe malaria; children with prostration should be observed closely and should receive parenteral antimalarial medication.

- Always exclude or, if in doubt, treat hypoglycaemia (see page 37).

- Seizures are common before or after the onset of coma and are significantly associated with morbidity and sequelae. Although many seizures present as overt convulsions, others may present in a more subtle way; important signs include intermittent nystagmus, salivation, minor twitching of a single digit or a corner of the mouth, an irregular breathing pattern and sluggish pupillary light reflexes.

- In children in profound coma, corneal reflexes and 'doll's eyes' movements may be abnormal.

- Abnormal motor posturing (Figure 4) is often observed in children with cerebral malaria, but the aetiology and pathogenesis are poorly understood: it may be associated with raised intracranial pressure and recurrence of seizures.

- In some children, extreme opisthotonus is seen (Figure 5), which may lead to a mistaken diagnosis of tetanus or meningitis.

- CSF opening pressure is usually raised (mean, 160mm) in children with cerebral malaria.

- Deep breathing (increased work of breathing generally, without signs of pulmonary consolidation) is a sensitive, specific sign of metabolic acidosis.

- Signs of impaired perfusion (delayed capillary refilling time > 2s, cool hands and/or feet or weak pulse) are common. Moderate hypotension (systolic blood pressure 70–80mm Hg) is present in 10% of children; however, severe shock (systolic blood pressure < 50mm Hg) is rare (< 2% of cases of severe malaria).

- Leukocytosis is not unusual in severe disease and does not necessarily imply an associated bacterial infection. This is also true in adults.

- Between 5% and 30% of children who survive cerebral malaria have some neurological sequelae, which may take the form of cerebellar ataxia, hemiparesis, speech disorders, cortical blindness, behavioural disturbances, hypotonia or generalized spasticity. Epilepsy is a sequela that develops in up to 10% of children, usually not until several weeks or months after the initial illness.

Management

- Institute emergency measures, including management of convulsions.

  - Some convulsions resolve spontaneously (within 5min), so no treatment other than supportive care is necessary

(ABC approach). Always set up an intravenous line and prepare medications. The most commonly available drug is diazepam; newer-generation benzodiazepines (e.g. midazolam, lorazepam) are associated with a lower incidence of respiratory depression.

– Wait 10min after giving diazepam. If the convulsions persist, give a second dose. Do not give more than two doses in 12h. Diazepam is poorly absorbed intramuscularly and should be given intravenously or rectally.

– If the convulsions persist after two doses of diazepam, give a loading dose of phenytoin or phenobarbitone if it is the only available option (see page 15). Check for respiratory depression and if present, provide ventilatory support.

• Prophylactic use of diazepam or any other anticonvulsant to prevent febrile convulsions is not recommended.

• Children with cerebral malaria may also have anaemia, respiratory distress (acidosis) and hypoglycaemia and should be managed accordingly.

– Check and treat for hypoglycaemia and hypoxia ($PaO_2 < 90\%$). If a pulse oximeter is not available, oxygen should still be given, especially for prolonged convulsions.

Figure 4: Motor posturing and possible seizure in a child with cerebral malaria.

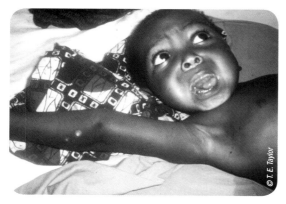

Note deviation of the eyes to the left (there was nystagmus), fixed grimace of the mouth and stereotyped raising of the arm

Figure 5: A child with cerebral malaria, exhibiting severe opisthotonic (extensor) posturing

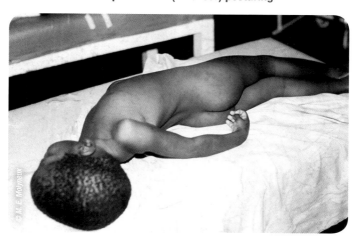

ANAEMIA

Severe anaemia is the leading cause of death in children with malaria.

Clinical features

Severe anaemia is a common presenting feature of falciparum and vivax malaria in areas of high transmission (Figure 6). It may result from repeated infections, in which case the asexual parasitaemia is generally low but there is abundant malarial pigment in monocytes and other phagocytic cells, reflecting recent or resolving infection. In chronic anaemia, physiological adaptation generally occurs, so that tachycardia and dyspnoea may be absent. Dyserythropoietic changes in the bone marrow are prominent.

Severe anaemia develops rapidly after infections with high parasite densities. In these cases, acute destruction of parasitized red cells is responsible for the anaemia, and careful monitoring during treatment is required. Children with acute onset of severe anaemia will not generally have had time to adapt physiologically and may present with tachycardia and dyspnoea. Anaemia may contribute to confusion and restlessness; signs of acidosis (deep breathing) and, very rarely, cardiopulmonary signs (cardiac failure), hepatomegaly and pulmonary oedema are seen.

Figure 6: Striking contrast between the palm of a child with anaemia, and that of his mother. Severe anaemia is the leading cause of death in children with malaria.

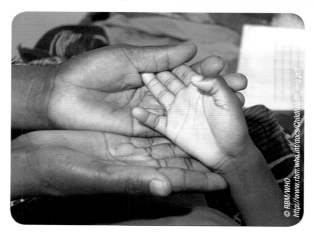

© RBM/WHO
http://www.rbm.who.int/docs/Childhealth_eng.pdf

Management

- The need for blood transfusion must be assessed with great care for each child. Not only erythrocyte volume fraction (haematocrit) or haemoglobin concentration but also the density of parasitaemia and the clinical condition of the patient must be taken into account.

- In general, in high-transmission settings, a haematocrit of ≤ 12% or a haemoglobin concentration of ≤ 4g/dl is an indication for blood transfusion, whatever the clinical condition of the child. In low-transmission settings a threshold of 20% haematocrit or a haemoglobin of 7g/dl, is recommended for blood transfusion (10ml of packed cells or 20 ml of whole blood per kg of body weight over 4h).

- In children with less severe anaemia (haematocrit of 13–18%, haemoglobin of 4–6g/dl), transfusion should be considered for those with any one of the following clinical features: respiratory distress (acidosis), impaired consciousness, hyperparasitaemia (> 20%), shock or heart failure.

- Anaemic children with respiratory distress are rarely in congestive cardiac failure. More commonly, their dyspnoea is due to acidosis, resulting from tissue hypoxia, often associated with hypovolaemia. The sicker the child, the more rapidly the transfusion must be given.

- A diuretic is usually not indicated, as many of these children are hypovolaemic. If, however, there is clinical evidence of fluid overload (the most reliable sign is an enlarged liver; additional signs are gallop rhythm, fine crackles at lung bases and/or fullness of neck veins when upright), furosemide (frusemide) at 1–2mg/kg of body weight up to a maximum of 20mg may be given intravenously.

- Follow-up of haemoglobin (haematocrit) levels after blood transfusion is essential. Many children require a further transfusion within the next few hours, days or weeks.

RESPIRATORY DISTRESS (ACIDOSIS)

Clinical features

Deep breathing, with indrawing (recession) of the bony structures of the lower chest wall, in the absence of localizing chest signs, suggests metabolic acidosis. Indrawing (recession) of the intercostal spaces alone is a less useful sign. Acidosis commonly accompanies cerebral malaria, severe anaemia, hypoglycaemia and features of impaired tissue perfusion. In many of these cases, respiratory distress is associated with an increased risk for death.

Management

- If the facilities are available, measure blood gases and arterial pH and continue to monitor oxygenation by oximetry.

- Correct any reversible cause of acidosis, in particular dehydration and severe anaemia. Intravenous infusion is best, at the most accessible peripheral site. If this is impossible, give an intra-osseous infusion (Annex 6). Take care not to give excessive fluid, as this may precipitate pulmonary oedema.

- If the haematocrit is < 18% or the haemoglobin concentration is < 6g/dl in a child with signs of metabolic acidosis, give screened whole blood (10ml/kg) over 30min and a further 10ml/kg over 1–2h without diuretics. Check the respiratory rate and pulse rate every 15min. If either shows any rise, transfuse more slowly to avoid precipitating pulmonary oedema.

- Monitor the response by continuous clinical observation supported by repeated measurement of acid–base status, haematocrit or haemoglobin concentration, and glucose, urea and electrolyte levels.

HYPOGLYCAEMIA

Clinical features

Owing to increased metabolic demands and limited glycogen stores, hypoglycaemia (blood glucose < 2.2mmol/l) is particularly common in children under 3 years especially those with anthropometric evidence of under-nutrition and in those with coma, metabolic acidosis (respiratory distress) or impaired perfusion. Mortality is increased with blood glucose levels < 2.2mmol/l. Hypoglycaemia should also be considered in children with convulsions or hyperparasitaemia. Hypoglycaemia is easily overlooked clinically because the manifestations may be similar to those of cerebral malaria (see also page 28). Children who are receiving a blood transfusion or who are not able to take oral fluids are at higher risk for hypoglycaemia and should be carefully monitored.

Management

- Hypoglycaemia (threshold for intervention, 3mmol/l) should be corrected with 500mg/kg of glucose. Using parenteral dextrose, immediately give 5ml/kg of 10% dextrose through a peripheral line, followed by a slow intravenous infusion of 5ml/kg per hour of 10% or 10ml/kg per hour of 5% to prevent recurrence of hypoglycaemia.

- If only 50% dextrose is available, dilute 1 volume of 50% dextrose with 4 volumes sterile water to get 10% dextrose solution (e.g. 0.4ml/kg of 50% dextrose with 1.6ml/kg of water for injection or 4ml of 50% dextrose with 16ml of water for injection). It is not recommended to give hypertonic glucose (> 20%) as it is an irritant to peripheral veins.

- If the intravenous route is not feasible, intra-osseous access (Annex 6) should be attempted. If this fails, give 1ml/kg body weight of 50% dextrose—or a sugar solution (4 level tea spoons of sugar in 200ml of clean water) through a nasogastric tube. Alternatively sugar may be given into the sublingual space. Check glucose levels after 30min. The duration and amount of dextrose infusion is dictated by the results of blood glucose monitoring (on blood taken from the arm opposite to that receiving the infusion), which can be done at the bedside with a glucometer, if available.

- Monitoring of blood glucose levels should continue even after successful correction, as hypoglycaemia may recur.

SHOCK

Clinical features

Signs of impaired perfusion are common (capillary refilling time > 2s, cool hands and/or feet). Moderate hypotension (systolic blood pressure < 70mm Hg in infants < 1 year and < 80mm Hg in children > 1 year) is present in 10% of cases, while severe hypotension (systolic blood pressure < 50mm Hg) is rare (< 2% of children with severe malaria).

Management

- Correct hypovolaemia with maintenance fluids at 3–4ml/kg per hour.

- Take blood for culture, and start the patient on appropriate broad-spectrum antibiotics immediately.

- Once the results of blood culture and sensitivity testing are available, check that the antibiotic being given is appropriate.

DEHYDRATION AND ELECTROLYTE DISTURBANCE

Clinical features

Severe dehydration (decreased skin turgor, intracellular volume depletion) may complicate severe malaria and may also be associated with signs of decreased peripheral perfusion, raised blood urea (> 6.5mmol/l; > 36.0mg/dl) and metabolic acidosis. In children presenting with oliguria and dehydration, examination of urine usually reveals a high specific gravity, the presence of ketones, low urinary sodium and normal urinary sediment, indicating dehydration rather than renal injury (which is rare in young children with malaria).

Hyperkalaemia (potassium > 5.5mmol/l) may complicate severe metabolic acidosis at admission. Hypokalaemia, hypophosphataemia and hypomagnesaemia are often apparent only after metabolic disturbances have been corrected after admission.

Management

- Children with severe dehydration should be given rapid IV rehydration followed by oral rehydration therapy. The best IV fluid solution is Ringer's lactate Solution (also called Hartmann's Solution for Injection). If Ringer's lactate is not available, normal saline solution (0.9% NaCl) can be used. 5% glucose (dextrose) solution on its own is not effective and should not be used. Give 100ml/kg of the chosen solution as follows: In children <12 months old give 30ml/kg bw in 1h, then 70ml/kg bw over the next 5h. While in children ≥12 months old, give 30ml/kg over 30mins, then 70ml/kg over next 2½h. Repeat the first dose of 30ml/kg if the radial pulse is still very weak or not detectable.

- After careful rehydration, acute kidney injury should be suspected if the urine output remains < 1ml/kg per hour (oliguria) and if urea and/or creatinine remain over the 95th centile for age.

- If acute renal injury is suspected and is complicated by signs of fluid overload (pulmonary oedema, increasing hepatomegaly), give furosemide intravenously, initially at 2mg/kg of body weight. If there is no response, double the dose at hourly intervals to a maximum of 8mg/kg of body weight (each dose should be given over 15min).

- Serial monitoring of plasma electrolytes is suggested; if abnormal values are detected, correction should be made according to international recommendations.

CHILDREN UNABLE TO RETAIN ORAL MEDICATION

Clinicians are often faced with ill children who do not meet the criteria for a diagnosis of severe malaria but who are unable to take or retain oral medication. As a delay in effective treatment for malaria may eventually result in severe malaria, such children should be admitted and treated with parenteral antimalarial agents or, when not possible, given pre-referral antimalarial treatment and referred to a centre where the appropriate supportive management can be provided until the child is able to tolerate oral medication.

POST DISCHARGE FOLLOW-UP OF CHILDREN WITH SEVERE MALARIA

Severe anaemia and neurological complications are important causes of mortality immediately after treatment for severe malaria. It is recommended that children be followed up on days 7, 14 and 28 (1 month) after discharge to monitor haemoglobin recovery. Persistent neurological sequelae will require a longer follow-up.

ANTIMALARIAL DRUGS

See the inside front cover flap and Annex 4.

Antimalarial drugs should be given parenterally for a minimum of 24h and replaced by oral medication as soon as it can be tolerated. Weigh the patient, and calculate the dose of malaria medicines according to body weight (mg/kg of body weight). For children, the recommended treatment is artesunate at 2.4mg/kg body weight given intravenously or intramuscularly at admission (time = 0), then at 12h, 24h, then once a day.

Artemether or quinine is an acceptable alternative if parenteral artesunate is not available: artemether at 3.2mg/kg body weight intramuscularly given at admission, then 1.6mg/kg body weight per day; or quinine at 20mg salt/kg body weight at admission (intravenous infusion or divided intramuscular injection), then 10mg/kg body weight every 8h; the infusion rate should not exceed 5mg salt/kg body weight per hour. Intramuscular injections should be given into the anterior thigh and *not* the buttock.

Do not attempt to give oral medication to unconscious children; if parenteral injection is not possible and referral is likely to be delayed, suppositories containing artesunate or any artemisinin should be administered as pre-referral treatment, while all efforts are made to transfer the child to a centre where appropriate care can be provided. If these routes are not possible, artemisinin-based combination therapy can be crushed and given by nasogastric tube. Nasogastric administration may, however, cause vomiting and result in inadequate drug levels in the blood.

CLINICAL FEATURES OF SEVERE MALARIA AND MANAGEMENT OF COMPLICATIONS IN ADULTS

In all cases of severe malaria, parenteral antimalarial chemotherapy should be started immediately and appropriate emergency measures and nursing care instituted. Any complications can then be dealt with as described below.

CEREBRAL MALARIA

Clinical features

Patients with cerebral malaria are comatose (for assessment of coma, see the Glasgow coma scale, Annex 5b). If the cause of the coma is in doubt, test for other locally prevalent causes of encephalopathy (e.g. bacterial, fungal or viral infection).

Asexual malaria parasites are nearly always demonstrable on a peripheral blood smear from patients with cerebral malaria. Convulsions and retinal changes (Figure 3) are common; papilloedema is rare. A variety of transient abnormalities of eye movement, especially dysconjugate gaze, have been described (Figure 7). Fixed jaw closure and tooth grinding (bruxism) are common. Pouting may occur, or a pout reflex may be elicited by stroking the sides of the mouth. Mild neck stiffness occurs, but neck rigidity and photophobia are absent. Motor abnormalities such as decerebrate rigidity and decorticate rigidity (arms flexed and legs stretched) occur. Hepatomegaly is common, but a palpable spleen is unusual. The abdominal reflexes are invariably absent; this is a useful sign for distinguishing hysterical adult patients with fevers due to other causes, in whom these reflexes are usually brisk. The opening pressure at lumbar puncture is usually normal (mean, 160mm) but is raised in 20% of cases; the CSF is usually clear, with fewer than 10 white cells per μl; protein may be slightly raised, as is the CSF lactate concentration. Computerized tomography or magnetic resonance imaging of the brain may show slight brain swelling attributable to increased cerebral blood volume.

Management

- Comatose patients should be given meticulous nursing care (see page 19).

- Insert a urethral catheter with a sterile technique.

- Insert a nasogastric tube, and aspirate the stomach contents.

- Keep an accurate record of fluid intake and output.

- Monitor and record the level of consciousness (on the Glasgow coma scale, Annex 5b), temperature, respiratory rate and depth, blood pressure and vital signs.

Treat convulsions if they arise with a slow intravenous injection of benzodiazepine (e.g. diazepam at 0.15mg/kg of body weight). Diazepam can be given intrarectally (0.5–1.0mg/kg of body weight) if injection is not possible. Patients with seizures that are not terminated by two doses of diazepam should be considered to have status epilepticus and given phenytoin (18mg/kg loading dose then a maintenance dose of 5mg/kg per day for 48h). If these are not available or fail to control seizures, phenobarbitone may be used (15mg/kg intramuscularly or a slow intravenous loading dose, then a maintenance dose of 5mg/kg per day for 48h). When phenobarbitone is used, monitor the patient's breathing carefully, as it can cause respiratory depression requiring ventilatory support. High-dose (20mg/kg) phenobarbitone has been shown to cause respiratory depression and an increased risk of death.

The following treatments for cerebral malaria are considered either useless or dangerous and should not be given:

- – corticosteroids and other anti-inflammatory agents
- – other agents given for cerebral oedema (urea, mannitol)
- – low-relative-molecular-mass dextran
- – epinephrine (adrenaline)
- – heparin
- – epoprostenol (prostacyclin)
- – cyclosporin (cyclosporin A)
- – deferoxamine (desferrioxamine)
- – oxpentifylline
- – large boluses of crystalloids or colloids

Figure 7: **Dysconjugate gaze in a patient with cerebral malaria: optic axes are not parallel in vertical and horizontal planes**

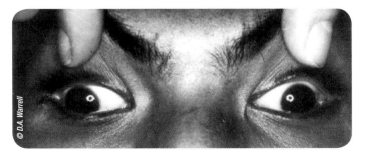

ANAEMIA

Clinical features

Anaemia is common in severe malaria and may be associated with secondary bacterial infection. Anaemia is a particularly important complication of malaria in pregnant women (see page 58).

Management

- If the erythrocyte volume fraction (haematocrit) falls below 20% or the haemoglobin concentration falls below 7g/dl, give a transfusion of screened, compatible fresh blood or packed cells (stored bank blood may be used if fresh blood is not available.)

- If necessary, give small intravenous doses of furosemide (frusemide), 20mg, during blood transfusion to avoid circulatory overload.

- Remember to include the volume of transfused cells or blood in calculating fluid balance.

ACUTE KIDNEY INJURY

Clinical features

Acute renal impairment (renal injury or failure) with raised serum creatinine and blood urea concentrations is an important manifestation of severe malaria, particularly in adults and older children. Although oliguria is usual, some patients maintain normal urine output despite rising blood urea and creatinine. Renal impairment may be part of multi-organ dysfunction in fulminant infections, which have a poor prognosis, or may follow recovery of other vital organ functions, in which case survival is usual if renal replacement can be maintained until the renal injury resolves. Renal injury in malaria is caused by acute tubular necrosis and is always reversible in survivors.

Management

- Exclude dehydration (hypovolaemia) by clinical examination, including measurement of jugular venous pressure (Annex 7), and the decrease in blood pressure between that taken when the patient is lying supine and that when he or she is propped up to 45°.

- If the patient is dehydrated, carefully infuse isotonic saline to correct hypovolaemia, monitoring the jugular venous pressure clinically with the patient propped up to 45°.

- If the patient remains oliguric after adequate rehydration and blood urea and creatinine continue to rise, then renal replacement therapy (haemofiltration or haemodialysis; if neither is available, peritoneal dialysis) may be required and should be implemented sooner rather than later, especially for acute fulminant disease.

- Haemofiltration is more efficient and is associated with a significantly lower mortality than peritoneal dialysis.

- Renal replacement therapy should be undertaken only in a centre with expertise to perform the procedure adequately and to provide the utmost care for the patient. When possible, refer the patient to a dialysis unit or centre.

HYPOGLYCAEMIA

Clinical features

Hypoglycaemia (blood glucose < 2.2mmol/l) is an important manifestation of falciparum malaria and is associated with an increased risk for mortality. It occurs in three groups of patients, which may overlap:

- patients with severe disease, especially young children;
- patients treated with quinine as a result of a quinine-induced hyperinsulinaemia; and
- pregnant women, either on admission or after quinine treatment.

In conscious patients, hypoglycaemia may present with classical symptoms of anxiety, sweating, dilatation of the pupils, breathlessness, a feeling of coldness, tachycardia and light-headedness. If the symptoms are protracted and severe, the patient may lose consciousness. Hypoglycaemia may precipitate generalized convulsions and extensor posturing.

Hypoglycaemia is easily overlooked because all these clinical features also occur in severe malaria itself. Deterioration in the level of consciousness may be the only sign. If possible, hypoglycaemia should be confirmed, ideally by a rapid test, especially in the high-risk groups listed above.

Management

- If hypoglycaemia (threshold for intervention, 3mmol/l) is detected by blood testing or suspected on clinical grounds, give 25g of dextrose (preferably as 10% dextrose) over a few minutes. Solutions of 50% and 25% dextrose are viscous and irritant and should not be used.

The usual dosage is 50ml of 50% dextrose (25 g) diluted with 100ml of any infusion fluid and infused over 3–5min.

- Follow with an intravenous infusion of 200–500mg/kg per hour of 5% or 10% dextrose.

- Continue to monitor blood glucose levels (with a rapid 'stix' method if available) in order to regulate the dextrose infusion. Remember that hypoglycaemia may recur even after treatment with intravenous dextrose.

METABOLIC ACIDOSIS

Metabolic acidosis is common in severe malaria and is an important cause of death. It is associated with hyperlactataemia. Low plasma bicarbonate is the single best prognosticator in severe malaria. Acidosis results primarily from microvascular obstruction by sequestered parasitized erythrocytes. The majority of adults with severe acidosis are not hypovolaemic, and, in those that are, rehydration often has no effect on the acidosis. In adults and older children, acidosis may result from acute renal failure. Acidosis commonly accompanies hypoglycaemia.

Clinical evidence of acidosis

Acidotic (Kussmaul) breathing is laboured, rapid, deep breathing. It commonly accompanies cerebral malaria, severe anaemia, hypoglycaemia and features of impaired tissue perfusion. In many of these cases, respiratory distress is associated with an increased risk for death. If the facilities are available, measure blood gases and arterial pH and continue to monitor oxygenation by oximetry.

Management

If there is evidence of dehydration:

- Give only isotonic fluid (0.9% saline) by slow intravenous infusion to restore the circulating volume, but avoid circulatory overload, which may rapidly precipitate fatal pulmonary oedema.

- Monitor blood pressure, urine volume (every hour) and jugular venous pressure (Annex 6).

- Improve oxygenation by clearing the airway, increasing the concentration of inspired oxygen and supporting ventilation artificially, if necessary.

PULMONARY OEDEMA

Clinical features

Pulmonary oedema is a grave complication of severe falciparum malaria, with a high mortality (over 80%); the prognosis is better in vivax malaria. Pulmonary oedema may develop several days after chemotherapy has been started, at a time when the patient's general condition is improving and the peripheral parasitaemia is falling. Pulmonary oedema in malaria has the features of acute respiratory distress syndrome, implying increased pulmonary capillary permeability. Pulmonary oedema may arise iatrogenically from fluid overload. The two conditions are difficult to distinguish clinically and may coexist in the same patient. Pulmonary oedema in falciparum malaria is often associated with other complications of malaria. The first indication of impending pulmonary oedema is an increase in the respiratory rate, which precedes the development of other chest signs (Figure 8). The arterial pO_2 is reduced. Hypoxia may cause convulsions and deterioration in the level of consciousness, and the patient may die within a few hours.

Figure 8: **Radiographic appearance of acute pulmonary oedema, resembling acute respiratory distress syndrome, in a patient with cerebral malaria**

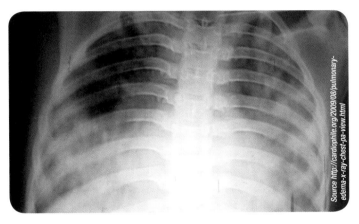

Source http://cardiophile.org/2009/08/pulmonary-edema-x-ray-chest-pa-view.html

Management

- Keep the patient upright; raise the head of the bed or lower the foot of the bed.

- Give a high concentration of oxygen by any convenient method, including mechanical ventilation.

- Give the patient a diuretic, such as furosemide (frusemide) at 0.6mg/kg (adult dose, 40mg), by intravenous injection. If there is no response, increase the dose progressively to a maximum of 200mg.

- In well-equipped intensive care units, mechanical ventilation with positive end-expiratory pressure and low tidal volume ventilation and a wide range of vasoactive drugs and haemodynamic monitoring will be available.

- If there is pulmonary oedema due to overhydration in addition to the above:
    - Stop all intravenous fluids and give furosemide.
    - If there is no improvement, withdraw 250ml of blood by venesection into a blood transfusion donor bag so that it can be given back to the patient later.
    - If there is renal impairment and no response to diuretics, use haemofiltration, if available.

SHOCK

Clinical features

Some patients are admitted in a state of collapse, with a systolic blood pressure < 80mm Hg (10.7kPa) in the supine position; cold, clammy, cyanotic skin; constricted peripheral veins; and a rapid, feeble pulse. This clinical picture may indicate complicating septicaemia, and possible sites of associated bacterial infection should be sought, e.g. meningitis, pneumonia, urinary tract infection (especially if there is an indwelling catheter) or intravenous injection site infection.

Patients with pulmonary oedema or metabolic acidosis or who have had massive gastrointestinal haemorrhage or ruptured spleen (a potential complication of *P. vivax* infection) may also present with shock. Dehydration with hypovolaemia may also contribute to hypotension.

Management

- Correct hypovolaemia with an appropriate plasma expander (fresh blood, plasma, dextran 70 or polyglycans). If these are not available, give isotonic saline.

- Take blood for culture, and immediately start the patient on appropriate broad-spectrum antibiotics.

- Once the results of blood culture and sensitivity testing are available, reassess the antibiotic treatment.

- Monitor jugular venous pressure (Annex 7).

ABNORMAL BLEEDING AND DISSEMINATED INTRAVASCULAR COAGULATION

Clinical features

Bleeding gums, epistaxis, petechiae and subconjunctival haemorrhages may occur occasionally. Disseminated intravascular coagulation, complicated by clinically significant bleeding, e.g. haematemesis or melaena, occurs in < 5% of patients. It is more common in low-transmission settings.

Management

- Transfuse fresh blood, clotting factors or platelets as required.

- Give vitamin K, 10mg, by slow intravenous injection.

- Start gastric protection with a parenteral histamine2-receptor blocker (e.g. ranitidine) or a proton pump inhibitor (e.g. omeprazole).

Thrombocytopenia is almost invariably present in falciparum malaria (black water fever), usually with no other coagulation abnormalities. In most cases, it is unaccompanied by bleeding and requires no treatment. The platelet count usually returns to normal after successful treatment of the malaria.

HAEMOGLOBINURIA

Clinical features

Haemoglobinuria is uncommonly associated with malaria. In adults, it may be associated with anaemia and renal impairment. Patients with glucose-6-phosphate dehydrogenase deficiency may develop intravascular haemolysis and haemoglobinuria precipitated by primaquine or other oxidant drugs, even in the absence of malaria.

Management

- Continue appropriate antimalarial treatment (see inside front cover flap) if parasitaemia is present.

- Transfuse screened fresh blood if necessary.

- If oliguria develops and blood urea and serum creatinine levels rise (i.e. if acute renal injury occurs), renal replacement therapy may be required. If possible, refer the patient to a dialysis unit or centre.

ANTIMALARIAL DRUGS

See inside front cover flap and Annex 4.

SPECIAL CLINICAL FEATURES AND MANAGEMENT OF SEVERE MALARIA IN PREGNANCY

SEVERE MALARIA

Clinical features

In moderate- and high-transmission settings, pregnant women, especially primigravidae, are susceptible to severe anaemia, but the other manifestations of severe malaria are unusual. Their malarial infection is often asymptomatic and may be overlooked because their peripheral blood films may be negative. Nonimmune pregnant women are at increased risk for severe falciparum malaria. Other signs suggestive of severe disease in these women, such as unconsciousness or convulsions, are more likely to be due to other causes, such as eclampsia or meningitis. Pregnant women with uncomplicated falciparum or vivax malaria have increased risks for abortion, stillbirth, premature delivery and low infant birth weight. Obstetric advice should be sought at an early stage; paediatricians should be alerted and the woman monitored closely. Blood glucose must be checked frequently, especially if the patient is on quinine.

Severe falciparum malaria is associated with substantially higher mortality in pregnancy than in non-pregnant women. Hypoglycaemia and pulmonary oedema are more frequent, and obstetric complications and associated infections are common. Severe malaria usually precipitates premature labour, and stillbirth or neonatal death is common. Severe malaria may also present immediately after delivery. Postpartum bacterial infection is a common complication in these cases.

Management

- Pregnant women with severe malaria should be transferred to intensive care if possible.

- Blood glucose should be monitored frequently.

- Obstetric help should be sought, as severe malaria usually precipitates premature labour.

- Once labour has started, fetal or maternal distress may indicate an intervention, and the second stage might have to be shortened by the use of forceps, vacuum extraction or caesarean section.

HYPOGLYCAEMIA

Clinical features (see page 48)

Hypoglycaemia may be present in pregnant women on admission or may occur after quinine infusion. It may be associated with fetal bradycardia and other signs of fetal distress. In severely ill patients, it is associated with lactic acidosis and high mortality.

In conscious patients who have been given quinine, abnormal behaviour, sweating and sudden loss of consciousness are the usual manifestations.

Management

- Treat as described on page 48. If the diagnosis is in doubt, 50% dextrose (20–50ml diluted and given intravenously) over 5–10min should be administered as a therapeutic trial.

- If injectable dextrose is not available, dextrose or sugar solution can be given to an unconscious patient through a nasogastric tube.

- Recurrent severe hypoglycaemia may be a problem in pregnant women.

PULMONARY OEDEMA

Clinical features

Pulmonary oedema may be present in pregnant women on admission, may develop suddenly and unexpectedly several days after admission or may occur immediately after childbirth (Figure 9).

Management

Treat as described on page 51.

Figure 9: **Acute pulmonary oedema developing immediately after delivery in a patient**

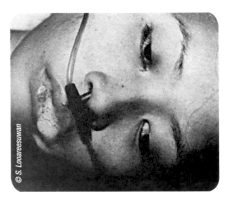

© S. Looareesuwan

ANAEMIA

Clinical features

Maternal anaemia is associated with maternal and perinatal morbidity and mortality and an increased risk for fatal postpartum haemorrhage. The malarial anaemia may be complicated by underlying iron and/or folic acid deficiency anaemia. Pulmonary oedema may develop in women who go into labour when severely anaemic or fluid-overloaded after separation of the placenta.

Management

- If the erythrocyte volume fraction (haematocrit) falls below 20% or the haemoglobin concentration falls below 7g/dl, give a transfusion of screened, compatible fresh blood or packed cells over 6h (with the precautions mentioned on page 46) and furosemide (frusemide) at 20mg intravenously.

- Folic acid and iron supplements may be required during recovery.

ANTIMALARIAL DRUGS

Parenteral antimalarial agents should be given to pregnant women with severe malaria at any stage of pregnancy, in full doses without delay. The rate of mortality from severe malaria in pregnancy is approximately 50%, which is higher than in non-pregnant women. Artesunate is the drug of choice. If this is not available, artemether is preferable to quinine in later pregnancy because quinine is associated with a 50% risk for hypoglycaemia.

PROGNOSTIC INDICATORS IN SEVERE FALCIPARUM MALARIA

The major indicators of a poor prognosis in children and adults with severe falciparum malaria are listed below.

Clinical indicators

- age < 3 years
- deep coma
- witnessed or reported convulsions
- absent corneal reflexes
- decerebrate or decorticate rigidity or opisthotonus
- clinical signs of organ dysfunction (e.g. renal injury, pulmonary oedema)
- respiratory distress (acidosis)
- shock
- papilloedema

Laboratory indicators

- hyperparasitaemia (> 250 000/µl or > 5%)
- peripheral schizontaemia
- peripheral blood polymorphonuclear leukocytosis (> 12 000/µl)
- mature pigmented parasites (> 20% of parasites)
- peripheral blood polymorphonuclear leukocytes with visible malaria pigment (> 5%)
- erythrocyte volume fraction (< 15%)
- haemoglobin concentration (<5g/dl)
- blood glucose < 2.2mmol/l (< 40mg/dl)

- blood urea > 60mg/dl
- serum creatinine > 265 µmol/l (> 3.0mg/dl)
- high CSF lactate (> 6mmol/l) and low CSF glucose
- raised venous lactate (> 5mmol/l)
- greater than threefold elevation in serum transaminases
- increased plasma 5'-nucleotidase
- raised muscle enzymes
- low antithrombin III levels
- very high plasma concentrations of tumour necrosis factor

COMMON ERRORS IN DIAGNOSIS AND MANAGEMENT

The common errors in the diagnosis and management of severe malaria are listed below.

ERRORS IN DIAGNOSIS

- failure to consider a diagnosis of malaria in a patient with either typical or atypical illness

- failure to elicit a history of exposure (travel history), including travel within a country with variable transmission

- misjudgement of severity

- failure to do a thick blood film

- failure to identify *P. falciparum* in a dual infection with *P. vivax* (the latter may be more obvious)

- missed hypoglycaemia

- failure to diagnose alternative or associated infections (bacterial, viral), especially in an endemic area with high transmission where *P. falciparum* and *P. vivax* parasitaemia may be 'incidental' rather than the cause of the illness

- misdiagnosis: making an alternative diagnosis in a patient who actually has malaria (e.g. influenza, viral encephalitis, hepatitis, scrub typhus)

- failure to recognize respiratory distress (metabolic acidosis)

- failure to conduct an ophthalmoscopic examination for the presence of papilloedema and malarial retinopathy

- misdiagnosis of severe *P. knowlesi* malaria. Mature stages of *P. knowlesi* are indistinguishable from *P. malariae*, and ring forms can resemble *P. falciparum*. For any patient from a knowlesi-endemic area with a microscopic diagnosis of *P. malariae*, treat with parenteral therapy if any features of severe malaria or parasitaemia > 100 000/ul. If testing for laboratory criteria for severe malaria is not readily available, treat with parenteral therapy if parasitaemia >20 000/ul.

ERRORS IN MANAGEMENT

- delay in starting antimalarial therapy this is the most serious error, as delays in starting treatment may be fatal.

- inadequate nursing care

- incorrectly calculated dosage of antimalarial medicines

- inappropriate route of administration of antimalarial agents (see inside front cover flap)

- intramuscular injections into the buttock, particularly of quinine, which can damage the sciatic nerve

- failure to switch patients from parenteral to oral therapy after 24h, or as soon as they can take and tolerate oral medication

- use of unproven and potentially dangerous ancillary treatment

- failure to review antimalarial treatment for a patient whose condition is deteriorating

- failure to re-check blood glucose concentration in a patient who develops seizure or deepening coma

- failure to recognize and treat minor ('subtle') convulsions

- failure to recognize and manage pulmonary oedema

- delay in starting renal replacement therapy

- failure to give antibiotics to treat possible meningitis presumptively if a decision is made to delay lumbar puncture

- fluid bolus resuscitation in children with severe malaria who are not severely dehydrated

ANNEX 1. SELECTED FURTHER READING

The WHO guidelines and manuals from which the recommendations in this manual were derived are:

Guidelines for the treatment of malaria, 2nd Ed. Geneva, World Health Organization, 2010. http://www.who.int/malaria/publications/atoz/9789241547925/en/index.html.

WHO pocket book of hospital care for children: guidelines for the management of common illnesses with limited resources. Geneva, World Health Organization, 2005.

Universal access to malaria diagnostic testing: an operational manual. Geneva, World Health Organization, 2011. http://whqlibdoc.who.int/publications/2011/9789241502092_eng.pdf.

Recommendations for the management of common childhood conditions: Evidence for technical update of pocket book recommendations. Geneva, World Health Organization, 2012. http://www.who.int/maternal_child_adolescent/documents/management_childhood_conditions/en/index.html.

ANNEX 2. MEMBERS OF THE REVIEW COMMITTEE

Technical Expert Group on Malaria Chemotherapy

Core members

Professor F. Binka (Co-chairman), School of Public Health, University of Ghana, Accra Ghana

Professor A. Björkman, Division of Infectious Diseases, Karolinska University Hospital, Stockholm Sweden

Professor M. A. Faiz, Department of Medicine, Sir Salimullah Medical College, Dhaka Bangladesh

Dr S. Lutalo, King Faisal Hospital, Kigali, Rwanda

Professor O. Mokuolu, Department of Paediatrics, University of Ilorin Teaching Hospital, Ilorin Nigeria

Professor N. White (Co-chairman), Faculty of Tropical Medicine, Mahidol University, Bangkok Thailand

Co-opted members

Professor N. Anstey, Menzies School of Health Research and Royal Darwin Hospital, Darwin Australia

Professor N. Day, Mahidol University, Bangkok, Thailand

Dr A. Dondorp, Faculty of Tropical Medicine, Mahidol University, Bangkok, Thailand

Prof. T. T. Hien, Hospital for Tropical Diseases, Ho Chi Minh City, Vietnam

Dr R. Idro, Department of Paediatrics and Child Health, Makerere University, Kampala, Uganda

Dr E. Juma, Division of Malaria Control, Ministry of Health, Nairobi, Kenya

Professor K. Maitland, KEMRI Wellcome Trust Programme, Kilifi, Kenya

Dr S. K. Mishra, Department of Internal Medicine, Ispat General Hospital, Rourkela, India

Professor M. Molyneux, College of Medicine, Malawi, and School of Tropical Medicine, University of Liverpool, UK

Dr G. Turner, Mahidol-Oxford Research Unit and Department of Tropical Pathology, Bangkok Thailand

Resource Persons

Dr Q. Bassat, Barcelona Centre for International Health Research (CRESIB) University of Barcelona, Hospital Clinic, Barcelona, Spain

Dr P. Kachur, Division of Parasitic Disease
and Malaria Center for Global Health
Centers for Disease Control and Prevention
(CDC), Atlanta, United States of America

WHO Secretariat

Dr A. Bosman, Global Malaria Programme,
WHO, Geneva, Switzerland

Dr M. Gomes, Special Programme for Research and
Training in Tropical Diseases, WHO, Geneva, Switzerland

Dr L. Muhe, Child and Adolescent Health and
Development, WHO, Geneva, Switzerland

Dr P. Olumese (Secretary), Global Malaria
Programme, WHO Geneva, Switzerland

Dr F. Pagnoni, Special Programme for Research and
Training in Tropical Diseases, WHO, Geneva, Switzerland

Dr P. Ringwald, Global Malaria Programme,
WHO, Geneva, Switzerland

Ms S. Schwarte, Global Malaria Programme,
WHO, Geneva, Switzerland

Dr M. Warsame, Global Malaria Programme,
WHO, Geneva, Switzerland

ANNEX 3. PERFORMING AND INTERPRETING RAPID DIAGNOSTIC TESTS

Rapid diagnostic tests (RDTs) can provide a diagnosis of malaria quickly in places where reliable microscopy is not possible or practical. RDTs detect antigens produced by malaria parasites and released into the blood; if the antigens are present, the test will be positive; if they are not, the test will be negative. Some antigens are produced by a single species of malaria parasite (e.g. *Plasmodium falciparum*), while some are produced by all malaria species (including *P. vivax, P. malariae, P. ovale* and *P. knowlesi*). The most widely used RDTs for detecting *P. falciparum* only target the HRP2 antigen, which is cleared relatively slowly; these RDTs may therefore be positive for several days after parasite clearance. This can be useful in testing patients with severe malaria who were pretreated with antimalarial agents and in whom parasitaemia has fallen below the level of microscope detection.

Requirements

To ensure reliable results with an RDT, the test kit and materials must be intact:

- a new RDT in unopened test pack with appropriate desiccant
- a new blood collecting device, provided in the RDT pack
- a new, unopened alcohol swab pack
- a new, unopened sterile lancet
- a new pair of disposable examination gloves

- buffer solution specific for the brand and batch of the RDT being used
- a watch or clock

RDT 1

Malaria Generic Pf RDT Results Guide

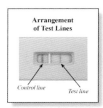

Arrangement of Test Lines

Control line   Test line

NEGATIVE RESULT

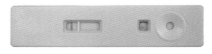

POSITIVE RESULTS

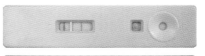

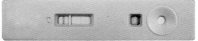

Plasmodium *falciparum*

Note: Test is positive even if the test line is faint.

INVALID RESULTS

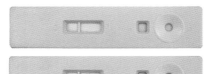

No Control Line

Note: Repeat the test using a new RDT if no control line appears.

RDT 2

Malaria Generic Pf-Pan RDT Results Guide

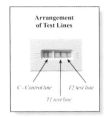

Arrangement of Test Lines

C - Control line | T2 test line
T1 test line

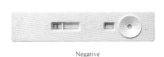

Negative

POSITIVE RESULTS

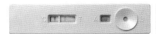

P. falciparum

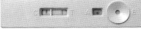

Non-falciparum (*P. vivax, P. ovale, P. malariae* or a mixed infection of these)

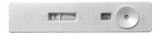

P. falciparum

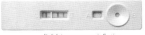

P. falciparum monoinfection or 'Mixed' Infection

NOTE: Test is positive even if the line in the test window is faint.

INVALID RESULTS

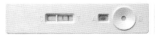

No Control Line

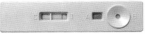

No Control Line

Repeat the test using a new RDT if no control line appears.

Note: Each test can be used **only once**.
Do not try to use the test more than once.

ANNEX 4. NOTES ON ANTIMALARIAL DRUGS

Artesunate

Current evidence indicates that artesunate is the drug of choice for the treatment of severe malaria. It is available in oral (in combination treatments), rectal and parenteral (injectable) formulations. When injected intramuscularly, artesunate is rapidly absorbed. Parasite clearance is faster than with quinine because artesunate kills young circulating ring-stage parasites. The drug is well tolerated, with no attributable local or systemic adverse effects. Rectal artesunate is the pre-referral treatment of choice for severe malaria, particularly in children; however, more studies are needed to clearly establish its effectiveness for pre-referral treatment in adults. Artemisinins can be used to treat pregnant women with severe malaria.

While oral artemisinin-based monotherapy is not recommended for the treatment of uncomplicated malaria because of the risks for relapse and for promoting the spread of artemisinin resistance, use of parenteral artesunate alone is standard for initial treatment of severe malaria in order to achieve rapid plasma therapeutic levels, which are not achieved as rapidly after oral administration. Furthermore, patients are usually initially unable to tolerate oral medication. All cases of severe malaria should be treated with a full course of a locally effective artemisinin-based combination medication once they are able to take oral medication and after at least 24h of parenteral therapy have been completed.

Artemether

Artemether is available in oral (in combination treatment), rectal and intramuscular formulations. Its efficacy, side-effects and availability are similar to those of artesunate, except that the parenteral formulation is oil-based and may be inadequately or erratically absorbed after intramuscular injection in severely ill patients.

Quinine

Intravenous quinine should always be given by rate-controlled infusion and never as a bolus ('push') intravenous injection. It may also be given intramuscularly into the anterior thigh (not the buttock) after dilution to 60–100mg/ml. While quinine commonly causes hypoglycaemia in pregnant women, it is safe for fetuses.

Mild side-effects are common, notably cinchonism (tinnitus, hearing loss, dizziness, nausea, uneasiness, restlessness and blurring of vision); serious cardiovascular and neurological toxicity is rare. Hypoglycaemia is the most serious and frequent adverse side-effect. In suspected quinine poisoning, activated charcoal given orally or by nasogastric tube accelerates elimination.

ANNEX 5. COMA SCALES

5A. BLANTYRE COMA SCALE FOR CHILDREN

The Blantyre coma scale[8] is modified from the widely used Glasgow coma scale[9] and is applicable to children, including those who have not learnt to speak.

Type of response	Response	Score
Best motor	Localizes painful stimulus[a]	2
	Withdraws limb from pain[b]	1
	Nonspecific or absent response	0
Verbal	Appropriate cry	2
	Moan or inappropriate cry	1
	None	0
Eye movements	Directed (e.g. follows mother's face)	1
	Not directed	0
Total		0–5

[a] Rub knuckles on patient's sternum or above patient's eyebrow.

[b] Firm horizontal pressure on thumbnail bed with a pencil

A state of unrousable coma is reached at a score of < 3. This scale can be used repeatedly to assess improvement or deterioration.

8   Molyneux ME et al. (1989). Clinical features and prognostic indicators in paediatric cerebral malaria: a study of 131 comatose Malawian children. *Quarterly Journal of Medicine*, 71:441–459.
9   Teasdale G, Jennett BJ (1974). Assessment of coma and impaired consciousness. A practical scale. *Lancet*, ii (7872):81–84.

5B. THE GLASGOW COMA SCALE
(FOR ADULTS AND CHILDREN > 5 YEARS)

Type of response	Response	Score
Eyes open	Spontaneously	4
	To speech	3
	To pain	2
	Never	1
Best verbal	Oriented	5
	Confused	4
	Inappropriate words	3
	Incomprehensible sounds	2
	None	1
Best motor	Obeys commands	6
	Purposeful movements to painful stimulus	5
	Withdraws to pain	4
	Flexion to pain	3
	Extension to pain	2
	None	1
Total		3–15

A state of unrousable coma is reached at a
score of <11. This scale can be used repeatedly
to assess improvement or deterioration.

ANNEX 6. SETTING UP AN INTRA-OSSEOUS INFUSION FOR CHILDREN

When intravenous access is impossible, an intraosseous infusion can be life-saving. It can be used to administer anything that would normally be given intravenously, i.e. fluids, whole blood, packed cells, glucose and medicines.

Requirements

- alcohol swabs

- a small syringe and fine needle for giving local anaesthetic (unnecessary if patient is comatose)

- an 18-gauge needle with trochar (special needles are made for intra-osseous infusion). Alternatively, a bone-marrow aspiration needle or even a standard 17–21-gauge disposable needle can be used, with care.

- an intravenous bottle and drip-set or a 50-ml syringe containing fluid for infusion

- local anaesthetic, e.g. 1% lidocaine or lignocaine

Procedure (with full sterile precautions)

- Choose a point for insertion of the infusion needle in the middle of the wide flat part of the tibia, about 2cm below the line of the knee joint (Figure A6.1).

- Do not use a site of trauma or sepsis.

- If the patient is conscious, infiltrate the skin and underlying periosteum with local anaesthetic.

- With the needle at right angles to the skin, press firmly with a slight twisting motion until the needle enters the marrow cavity with a sudden 'give'.

- Attach a 5-ml syringe, and aspirate to confirm that the position is correct. The aspirate can be used for blood films, blood culture and blood glucose measurement.

- The infusion needle should be held in place under sticking plaster (or a plaster of Paris cast, as with a scalp vein infusion) and the child's mother or carer entrusted with holding the leg.

- You can place an infusion in each leg, either simultaneously or in sequence, if necessary.

- An alternative site for an intra-osseous infusion is the antero-lateral surface of the femur, 2–3cm above the lateral condyle.

- An infusion allowed to drip through the needle in the usual way (by gravity) may go very slowly. For urgent administration, use a 50-ml syringe to push in the required fluid in boluses.

Possible complications

Sepsis. Do not leave an intra-osseous line in one site for more than 6–8h. After this time, sepsis is increasingly likely.

Compartment syndrome. If the needle is allowed to pass entirely through the tibia, fluid may be infused into the posterior compartment of the leg, causing swelling and eventually impairing circulation. Check the circulation in the distal leg at intervals.

Figure A6.1 Site for insertion of intra-osseous infusion in the tibia

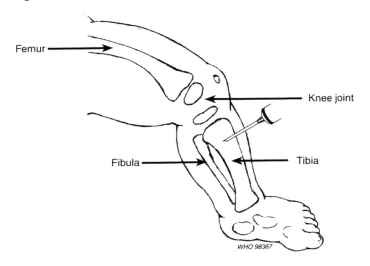

ANNEX 7. MEASURING JUGULAR VENOUS PRESSURE

Jugular venous pressure is a clinical measure of central venous pressure (Figure A7.1). It is the height of the pulsating column of blood in the great veins draining into the right atrium. Its value in malaria is in assessing fluid replacement treatment of over- or underhydration (hyper- or hypovolaemia). Nevertheless, the relation between central venous pressure and the effective blood volume is highly variable in severe malaria.

The jugular venous pressure is the vertical distance, measured in centimetres, between the venous pulsation in the neck and the sternal angle (junction of the second rib with the sternum) when the patient is propped up on pillows at 45° to the horizontal. In this position, the sternal angle marks the level of the right atrium. The height of jugular venous pressure is normally 4–5cm. In order to measure it, the patient should be made as comfortable and relaxed as possible, as it is difficult or impossible to identify venous pulsation if the neck muscles are contracted. Try to achieve good (oblique) lighting of the neck. Look for the jugular venous pulse in the internal jugular vein or its external jugular tributaries on both sides of the neck with the patient's chin tilted up and slightly away from you.

Certain characteristics help to distinguish jugular venous pulsation from carotid arterial pulsation. The jugular venous pulse:

- has two waves for each carotid artery pulsation. Make this comparison by gently palpating the carotid pulse on the opposite side of the neck.

- falls with inspiration and rises with expiration (except where there is cardiac tamponade);

- can be obliterated by pressing firmly but gently with the back of the index finger placed horizontally just above the clavicle at the root of the neck;

- may be visible only when the patient is lying flat (in cases of hypovolaemia) or sitting upright at 90° (for example, in severe congestive cardiac failure); and

- is usually impalpable.

Do not be misled by what appears to be high venous pressure but is just a non-pulsatile column of blood trapped in the external jugular vein. To double-check, press firmly and gently just above the clavicle so as to trap blood in the external jugular veins. When the pressure is suddenly released, the engorged veins should collapse immediately unless there is high central venous pressure. The jugular venous pressure cannot be assessed when there is gross tricuspid valve regurgitation.

Figure A7.1 Measurement of the height of the jugular venous pressure

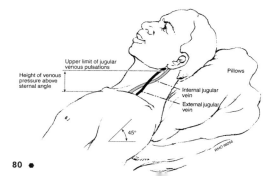

ANNEX 8. PERITONEAL DIALYSIS

Peritoneal dialysis (Figure A8.1) is inferior to haemofiltration in renal replacement but may be the only option in some settings. It can be used to manage acute renal failure in severe malaria. Peritoneal dialysis has three phases: *fill*, in which dialysate is introduced into the abdomen; *dwell*, 4–6h during which the dialysate remains in the abdomen; and *drain*, when the dialysate is drained by gravity.

Requirements
- Tenckhoff peritoneal catheter
- tubing and a Y-connector
- drainage bag
- dialysate (dialysis fluid)
- local anaesthetic
- lancet
- sutures
- sterile dressings

Procedure

Using aseptic technique, clean and drape the abdomen. With the area under local anaesthetic, make an infraumbilical incision into the abdomen and introduce a Tenckhoff peritoneal catheter or any soft multi-perforated catheter. Close the incision, secure the catheter and apply a sterile dressing. Connect the catheter through a Y-connector with one end of the Y in the dialysate bag and another in a drainage bag. Warm the dialysate to body temperature. Initially, run it into the drainage bag to clear air from the tubing and prevent its introduction into the abdominal cavity.

Use an appropriate amount of dialysate for the age, size and condition of the patient. Do not overfill the abdomen, which will compromise respiration. The frequency of cycling depends on the patient's condition and response.

Monitoring

Fluid input and output, temperature, pulse, respiration, blood electrolytes and glucose, and the clarity of the dialysate must be monitored regularly. A cloudy dialysate is indicative of peritonitis.

Possible complications

Peritonitis, bowel perforation, lung-base collapse (atelectasis), pneumonia, pulmonary oedema, hyperglycaemia (dialysate contains dextrose), hypovolaemia, hypervolaemia and adhesions are possible complications.

Figure A8.1 Illustration showing peritoneal dialysis

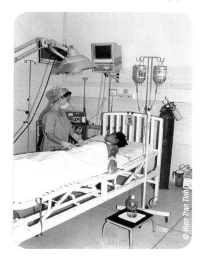

ANNEX 9. CALCULATING VOLUMES OF MAINTENANCE FLUIDS AND BLOOD TRANSFUSIONS

Maintenance fluids

Weigh the patient and calculate the volume of maintenance fluids as follows:

- 4ml/kg body weight per hour for the first 10kg

- 2ml/kg body weight per hour for the next 10kg

- 1ml/kg body weight per hour for weight above 20kg

  On the basis of this example, the volume of maintenance fluids for a:

  - 7kg child is 7x 4 =28ml/hour,

  - 20kg child is (10x4) +(10x2)= 60ml/hour, and

  - 28kg child is (10x4) + (10x2) + (8x1) =68ml/hr.

- Add quantified fluid losses.

- Add 10–15% for every degree in temperature above 38°C.

Transfusion volume for children with severe anaemia [10]

Weight in kg

Increment in haemoglobin (Hb; g/dl) is the desired Hb – current Hb

Haematocrit expressed as a decimal, e.g. haematocrit of 20 = 0.2

$$\text{Blood volume} = \frac{\text{Weight (kg) x increment in Hb (g/dl) x 3}}{\text{Haematocrit}}$$

10 Davies P et al. (2007). Calculating the required transfusion volume in children. *Transfusion*, 47:212–216.